Cover Page

EXERCISE HABITS

EXERCISE HABITS

The Daily Exercise Habits Affordable To Help You Change Your Life And Achieve Freedom And Wellness

Stephen-Jones Johnson

Other Books By
Stephen-Jones Johnson

Self-Confidence

The Self-Love Mastery

To William.

I love You So Much.

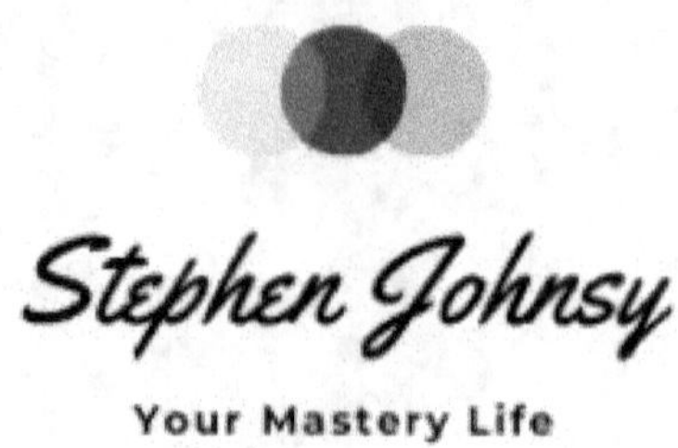

Stephen Johnsy
Your Mastery Life

Table of Contents

ACKNOWLEDGEMENTS

My very deepest thanks to all those who have helped me, directly or indirectly throughout this journey and climb all the mountains to be here today:

William, Evie, Thandie, Kelly, Helen, Tshiamo, Patrick & Christina Ndongo, Innocent and Erica. Thank you for your continued support and inspiration.

I have met a lot of amazing individuals whom we've shared so much over the years and I wish I could mentioned all of you here but if I do we'll be here for the long haul... So I thank you for being who you are and for teaching me a thing or two. Most importantly, thank you for being in my life.

INTRODUCTION

I want to thank you and congratulate you for purchasing this book, "Exercise Habits".

This book contains proven and evidence based steps and strategies on how to Make Exercise A Habit. Through these evidence based steps and strategies you'll be able to reach your goals, change your life and achieve your freedom and wellness you've longed for.

This book gives you the steps you can easily use to help yourself start living a healthy active lifestyle on daily basis as a habit. It will also allow you to see that exercising can be fun and enjoyable at the same time.

You will be able to see the need to take the first step that will lead you taking control of your life.

Below is a brief preview of what you'll learn from reading this book:

- How to make a commitment and stick with it to the end

- Why habits are important

- How to best achieve your desire goal

- How to overcome the challenges you'll face

- Maintaining your progress through the entire journey

- Approaches on how to build the exercise habit

- How to become accountable for your actions

- How good nutrition is important for your success

- To finally plan and enjoy the life you deserve

- And many more

So take action right away to begin your journey to Wellness and Freedom while having fun every day by reading this book.

Once again thank you for purchasing this book, I hope you enjoy it!

...

CHAPTER 1

Background

"Purpose is the reason for Your Journey. Passion is the fire that lights up the journey" ~ Unknown

How many habits do you have?

If you stop to think about it, you probably have dozens, maybe even hundreds, of habits. Not all of them are good habits of course. Some habits, like cursing or drinking sugary soda, are not great for you. How did you acquire those habits – the good and the bad ones?

Did you decide to make them habits or did they just happen?

For your bad habits, chances are they just sort of happened. One Coke at lunchtime turned into a daily regular thing and it grew from there.

Good habits happen this way as well. Good habits can also be created deliberately and with intention. For example, you might have taken the stairs the first day of work, and ever since then you've always taken the stairs instead of the elevator.

Habits are important because they are said to take the guesswork and the thinking out of the process. For example, brushing your teeth could be considered a habit. You brush them every morning and probably every night. Do you think "Should I brush my teeth?" or does it happen pretty automatically? It's probably fairly automatic for most people.

The exercise habit can be like that as well. It can be automatic so that you don't have to think, "Should I exercise?" You just do it.

What Is A Habit

As you probably know, a habit is a routine of repeated behaviours that we do regularly and consistently as part of our daily lives. Psychology Today has emphasised the findings that these repeated behaviours can be difficult to change because they're "literally etched into our neural pathways," which can be a challenge when you want to change the behaviour or start a new habit.

Mind you, a habit can be bad and can also be good depending on what it is. The great news though, is that these etched patterns especially the bad ones can be changed over time with certain measure put in place.

One of the interesting strategy to help you with this is stated in the book by Charles Duhigg called "The Power of Habit" where he talks about the concept of the Habit Loop to help you understand how the habit is formed with reiteration on the three elements: the cue (trigger), he behaviour(routine) and the reward(benefit). I recommend this book for you to check it out.

As you now know, the reason you haven't been successful in sticking to your exercise regime is not that you can't do it. It's because the things you have in place or your distractors have been there for a long time and the only way to overcome them is by re-wiring your brain pathways again. They're different examples I can use here, I am sure you have a lot too; but I will use the one I do every day.

I put out my gym clothes the night before and put them where I can see them when I wake (Cue). When I get up , the first thing I do is get into my gym clothes and prepare myself to head-out to the gym to perform my session for that day (Routine). Finally after completing my session and getting back home, I feel great and/or I see my results and the feeling is amazing, I can then treat myself with something nice I like (Reward).

LET'S BE HONEST THOUGH, embarking on an exercise journey and even remaining consistent can be a challenge and finding ways to make it more easier can be the best solution.

However, for it to become more easier and for you to achieve those goals you have, you have to find routines that you can do daily and consistently to be able to make it a habit.

I must mention also that as we are all different, some people have different habit building personalities. Some love to schedule, while others resist the calendar.

Some people love tracking results, while others despise any sort of quantitative analysis of their lifestyle. Some prefer to dive in as they are inspired by large, seemingly impossible, goals. While others prefer to take it step by step. Whatever your preferred way is, go with that because you want to be engaged in something that you enjoy and will be able to maintain throughout.

I am sure you may relate to this as we have all done it so many times; you've started a new exercise routine and really loving it – you're focused, motivated, committed and you can't wait to get up and head to the gym or have a run each morning!!! But then, you stop or slowly your passion drops until you don't want to do it, WHY? What is causing this decline in interest or passion.

Usually within a few days or weeks those good intentions disappear because we throw in the towel so early especially if we don't see the results soon enough. Maybe it's because one didn't prepare well enough for the long haul or the challenges that comes with starting something new. Most of us usually think we fail because of lack of motivation to keep going, but that is not necessarily the truth.

What has been identified as the main reason why people fall is the fact that there was no plan from the beginning, a long term one which would allow the habit to form and make it easy to keep going. There is no plan for when the challenges arise, or when self-doubt kicks in!

The question now is, how do you keep up and what is the best way to help yourself remain consistent and persevere on a daily basis? There are a few ways in which one can adopt in order to reach their fitness goals and remain consistent.

It all starts with a decision you first make of wanting to improve yourself. Then you have to make that commitment by taking the first step to actually starting your journey and hopefully staying on course till the end! If you believe that you can do it, have confidence in yourself and the plan in place, there is no reason as why you can't make it.

Before you going forward, you might want to hear this as it will help you in some way to find what works for you. Several studies have been conducted to find out what was the major motivating factor for those who started the journey, persevered through it all and never looked back to achieve their results. The studies showed that they succeeded because the following kept them going: Appearance, Feeling of Well-being, Weight management, Love of exercise, Sleeping better, Doing Something they enjoyed, Productivity in their life increased and also by just making Self-care a priority.

Starting a new habit can be a challenge and maintaining it is not the sexiest topic if we are honest! That is why you have to have your strong reasons to keep to keep going. As mentioned above, when you have a strong reason to keep going, you will always find a way to help you achieve your goal. You must become your biggest cheerleader because you will encounter challenges and if you're not strong mentally, you will give up. This is the key to achieving your results and living a healthy active lifestyle.

Numerous studies have been done to prove that when certain habits are adopted and maintained, individuals are nudged to keep going and achieve their desired results. Below are the top tips that can help you cement your exercise routine into your life and make it a habit and part of your daily healthy active lifestyle.

Remember that it takes time to plan, arrange and set everything in motion for you to start a new habit, so give yourself that time to organise everything. A thorough planning especially if you're planning on losing weight is what will help you win in the long run.

PROVEN TIPS TO HELP You Make Exercise A Habit

One thing I totally agree with is the idea of doing your exercises daily! I know you're probably thinking, what? daily? Yes, daily but just to clarify, this doesn't mean you have to go to the gym every day! There are different ways in which you can do your exercises as you will find below.

Whatever you choose to adopt as your main exercise has to be something you can afford to do and be consistent with. A walk, a swim, gym workouts, a run, play ball, all these are great ways to get your body moving. Remember the main thing is for you to be able to do it regularly.

If you're interested and committed to achieving your fitness goals (or any other goals), you will always find a way to the summit. Obviously it'll not be easy, but your mindset will help you get there. So indulge yourself and learn something below, you can do it!

CHAPTER 2

Set Realistic and Reasonable Goals

Having a goal that you're working towards can be a powerful motivator. Losing weight or getting into shape are good goals in theory, but they're big-picture goals that need perseverance and consistency. So you have to start thinking small and slowly get your way up. At the same time, you don't want to be stagnant in your journey so you should slowly push yourself to do a little extra each time.

As we always say, nothing worth having is meant to come easy, there will be change and sometimes even pain! But it's all part of the package to get where you want to be. The great thing is that you'll get there if you persevere. The catch is that the goal has to be something you can reasonably attain, your big 'WHY' that you believe you can reach.

Are you familiar with the term SMART goals? It's an acronym that stands for Specific, Measurable, Attainable, Relevant, and Time-Sensitive. Some people thrive on this type of goal setting method, but to be honest, regardless of your habit formation personality it's a good idea to consider these elements as they'll help you on your journey. Let's take a quick look at each letter individually so it make sense.

SPECIFIC

What EXACTLY do you want to achieve? Do you want to lose 30 pounds, exercise for 30 minutes a day, or reach a deadlift PR of 200 pounds? Many people approach exercise habits like this; "I just want to exercise every day" or "I want to lose weight." This approach doesn't work. You have to figure out what you want so that you can create a path to achieve it.

You have to be specific. So close your eyes and imagine your goal. What do you want your life to look like? What specific exercise habit do you want to create?

Keep in mind that it might be a bit complicated. "I want to strength train, do cardio, and some yoga" could turn into "I want to strength train twice a week, do cardio three times a week, and yoga twice a week." From there, you can build a plan and a habit.

Measurable

This is simple enough; how can you quantify your habit? Distance, time, and frequency are all measurable. Run for 30 minutes, ride your bike for 15 miles, run for 30 minutes, exercise five days a week, etc.

Attainable

Your goal must be something that's possible. For example, running a marathon tomorrow or losing 100 pounds next week are not attainable goals. Running a marathon in a few months or losing 100 pounds in a year are attainable – with a good habit and plan.

Relevant and Time-Sensitive

Relevant simply means that your goal must relate to the habit that you want to cultivate and achieve.It has to be something that you know you can be consistent with.

Time-sensitive isn't applicable to all goals. However, often if there's a time limit, it makes it easier to create a plan. For example, "I want to run a marathon in six months," or "I want to lose 60 pounds by January." The time limit helps you focus on your habit.

So goals are a part of many successful habits, but they're not the only element of success as you will know from this book, especially when we're talking about exercise habits so let's continue.

Some questions to ask yourself when setting goals are like; is this something I can be consistent with? Does it align with and make sense for my big-picture goals? Will it get me the results I'm after or bring me closer to those results? Do I enjoy it?

Make Commitment For A Month

For starters, commit yourself to at least four weeks of exercise regime. The idea here is that by the time you complete this, the new habit would be pretty much engraved in you. This has been proven as well in a randomised control study done by Milkman and her colleagues at Wharton School of Business. They found that those participants who joined a four weeks challenge were more likely to continue with their new habit for up to ten months!

They make an important point that the "key to habits is repetition. And if you can get that repetition going while you have high motivation, you're likely to have a behaviour change that lasts."

While making this commitment, decide when is the best time to suit you and your new habit, whether in the morning or evening. You know yourself better, so use the time that you know you're at your most productive. Schedule it in and make it a non-negotiable time, have that time blocked on your calendar. If you put it on the calendar and make time for it, it will happen. It's like adding it to the calendar means it's a priority. You do it without thinking about it because it's on your schedule.

Maybe think about how you organise your life right now. Are you a scheduler? Do you live by your calendar? For example, Maryna likes to schedule everything because it works for her. She schedules when she checks her email. She schedules household chores, lunch, work time, appointments, and yes, she schedules her exercise as well. It works for her and help her to stay focused and offers her the structure she needs. Each "Appointment" is tended to because it's on her calendar. If this sounds like you, consider embracing this habit forming approach and see what happens.

Remember, you're trying to become the best version of yourself and achieve your goal so you have to stay committed to this. Obviously urgent things do come up, disrupt out schedule and it's okay that part of life. The important thing is that you fin another way and juggle a bit to accommodate that but remember why you started.

CHAPTER 3

Do Something You Enjoy

There nothing better and fulfilling than doing something that you enjoy! As mentioned earlier, daily exercise doesn't mean lifting heavy weights every day. What you want to do is something that you'll enjoy, manage and afford to do regularly. Something that brings excitement within you when you think about it. It has been proven that when you bundle up your passion with some form of exercise or something healthy, you're bound to do it more often.

What you don't want to do is associate your new habit with pain, so it is important to start with something easy to do and slowly improve yourself. As with anything new, you want to start slowly, learn the trick and tips on how to become better at it. Once your confidence has set it, you can push to another gear to challenge yourself.

The most common reason why people don't succeed in achieving their fitness goals is that when they think about exercise, don't think that it's fun. Exercise for them is something that they feel they're supposed to do, it's a chore. It's like taking your vitamins or eating your veggies. You may not love it but you do it because you're supposed to. That's not the way it has to be.

You can maybe try looking back at what you used to enjoy. What did you love to do as a child? If nothing comes to mind, then look forward. What have you always wanted to try? What looks like it might be fun?

For example, regular walks after dinner, yoga, boxing or rock climbing might look like something fun to try. What about ballroom dancing or fencing? Exercise doesn't necessarily mean lacing up your running shoes and hitting the treadmill or elliptical for an hour. It can mean that if you want it to. But there's nothing wrong with doing any form of exercise that gets your body moving, that should be the main aim. If you're motivated by fun and want to add more fun to your day, then consider looking for movements and activities that work your body and bring a smile to your face. You may find that the exercise habit is the easiest thing you've ever done for yourself.

There is nothing exciting and fulfilling than seeing yourself do things you couldn't do before! It gives you the best joy as you see your hard work paying off.

Get Yourself A New Workout Outfit

This may sound strange because some people think gym clothes don't matter! But they couldn't be further from the truth. You definitely want to workout on clothes that fit you well and make you feel comfortable. Whether it's the colour or design of the clothes, it matters most; it helps you have that confidence because you feel good about yourself.

One thing to remember though is that you're at the gym or wherever you do your exercise to work on yourself to get the best results you can. Everyone started somewhere so don't be intimidated by those who are already ahead of you. If you're not confident yet to start your journey at your gym, start at home to build yourself and yes, you still have to get new workout wear, it acts a motivator.

Give yourself the time you need but at some point you have to face the challenge of being at the gym seeing a lot of other people. You'll be surprised at how much you learn there and what results you get!

Find Your Exercise Buddy

Accountability is a strong motivator for some. The word "accountable" means that you're responsible for your actions. Of course we're all responsible for our actions and non-actions, but for some it takes a little extra accountability to help create a habit. For example, signing up for a gym membership is a form of accountability. The monthly payments and the expense can help hold you accountable. Some people tend to be motivated when they're accountable to someone else. There are actually a few ways that you can leverage this to help you create an exercise habit.

It's very important to find a workout partner who will keep you accountable. This will help you stay on track and be motivated to actually leave your house. You can set a specific time with your friends for your exercises so you can keep each other accountable.

The social aspect of having a buddy is huge because when you've agreed to go a run or walk etc. you don't want to disappoint your buddy and this lead to you getting over those excuses you initially had.

Do you have a child, sibling, or friend who needs a boost and a bit of motivation to exercise? There are some personalities that find it's easier to create a habit if they are able to take on the status of a role model. You're accountable to the person that you're trying to help out.

For example, your child joins the track team and needs to practice on their own. You want to start your own running exercise habit. By being a role model to your child, you can join them on their practice runs and achieve your own exercise habit goals.

Accountability doesn't work for everyone. However, it can be a significant resource if it suits your habit forming personality.

Make your exercise a non-negotiable routine that your family knows and accept that you do. Tell them of your workout buddies and when the scheduled times are. This will is important so they can support you and not try to discourage you every time you go for it. This can play a major role in you achieving your results.

CHAPTER 4

Do Not Restrict Yourself

The idea is to help you remain consistent with your new habit, so do not restrict yourself with the same exercises every day and at the same time. It becomes monotonous and boring and you might end up losing interest. It has been proven that when you become flexible with your exercise routine and mixing it a little bit, you're bound to get more results.

This also allows you to target different muscle groups each time you do a different exercise from the day before. You're also allowing the other muscles time to recover and grow! Recovery is actually the most important time phase as it'll help give you the results you want.

Make A Commitment To Yourself

Here's the thing, there are going to be days when going to the gym and working out is going to be the last thing you want to do. It happens to all of everyone. The important thing is not to fall victim to that and start skipping your sessions. Try by all means not to skip any day but if you do, don't beat yourself up and feel bad. We all do mess up sometimes, however, what matters most is how we recover from that setback!

IF YOU HAVE FALLEN down, get yourself together and rise up again because you have a goal to reach. Remember that consistency is an important key to your success. Never let any obstacles dictate your end results! If you think you're struggling, get an accountability partner who will help and motivate you to keep going.

Research shows that if you plan a session with a buddy of yours, you're more likely to turn up for the session. That's is why people who join a challenge are more likely to succeed.

Nowadays we have a lot of online fitness challenges that are just as effective, it's a community that will support you. Once you start, you never want to stop because the community is supportive of each other.

I was skeptical when I started, the benefits I got were beyond what I had in my mind and I have never looked back. Now I can't imagine my life without physical activity and a daily healthy active lifestyle. You build social networks through these programs and your life is never the same!

Record Your Progress and Take Pictures

Sometimes it may look like you're not progressing at all and it's fine because progress takes time. However, it is so important to take your before photo and keep it safe, why? because this will reward you later when you compare with your progress photo. Photo and video of your workout do help you see your journey. Get in the habit of logging in what's important to you during your exercises or trainings.

This usually helps when you later look at where you have come from.

I bet you'd be tempted to look in the mirror every day for new results but it can be hard to notice any change especially if you're doing it daily. But keeping your photos allows you to actually see that change because if you're working hard and following the plan, there is no reason why you can't' get your results.

But beyond the physical results, there are more other amazing benefits of daily physical activity which when you see them, will definitely be motivated. Think of things like; more energy or a better mood throughout the day, better sleep patterns, clothes fitting better, a decrease in stress levels, performance in the gym getting better, etc. Take note of these things so you can see how your progress over time has been.

CHAPTER 5

Ensure You Have A Rest Day

One thing to never take for granted is having a rest day. Your recovery is as much important as your daily workout, so set a day that suits you and get some rest. My rest day is Sunday, not matter what happens I never workout on Sunday. If you're a beginner and your workouts are about twenty minutes in length, then maybe you can go without a rest day. Whatever the case, do what works well for you but I still want to emphasise the importance of letting your body rest.

It is however still I good idea to rest from your usual exercises. Resting your body allows your muscles the chance to fully recover and for growth to take place as well. Remember you want to make the experience pleasurable and make it a daily habit. So by not resting enough, you're predisposing yourself to associating the habit with pain, and that will lead to your downfall.

Better Nutrition Better Life

Your health is the cornerstone of your wellbeing and healthy eating habits will determine how you live your life, either with or without any restrictions. Several studies have shown that when you improve your habits in certain areas of your life, it causes a ripple effects as a result and you become better in other areas you were not even focusing on. That's great isn't it!

You have probably heard of the eighty twenty rule where your nutrition takes up eighty percent and the remaining twenty percent taken by exercise. This allows you to adapt well into the new routine of your exercises while getting enough and proper nourishment to the body for optimal results.

This is why consistency is very important so you can give the body a chance to adapt to your new regime of both nutrition and exercise habits. Achievement of your goals all stems from following both these ideas to allow that new habit to form and be engrained in you. So wherever possible, try to eat a healthy balance meal, involve a health or wellness coach or even a dietician if you have to.

Someone once said "Your health is Your Wealth" and it's absolutely true, as I'm the testament of that and you can be too!

Reward Yourself

You may be thinking what? - the reward is for the results at the end of your goal achievement! Well, that's not entirely good enough because you need something to keep you going as you're headed towards your goal.

The key to making a reward-based exercise habit work is to make sure that:

A) You don't just skip the habit and buy yourself the reward anyway

B) The reward is actually motivating for you

C) The exercise habit is one that you can realistically achieve. Just because you're rewarding yourself doesn't mean you have to create an exercise routine that's near impossible to follow through on

If you're not sure if a reward-based exercise habit would work for you, start by imagining your day with a reward-based habit. What would you reward yourself with? It can be anything from a relaxing book and a bath at the end of the day if you exercise, to a vacation if you exercise five days a week for three months. Clothing, outings, and even a day off from work and responsibilities can be exciting and motivating rewards as well.

It has been proven by the study published by Sport, Exercise and Performance Psychology that when you reward yourself as you go, you increase and strengthen your desire to work out. This will lead you to building that habit to keep going for your goal.

You can buy yourself some new running or walking shoes after you've achieved one month of consistency on your journey. You can buy yourself a book to read or music album or go and see a play, just find something that make you happy and look forward to next reward for working hard on yourself.

CHAPTER 6

Your Mindset Is Key

Like anything we do in life, there are challenges that comes with it and starting a new fitness routine is no different. You will encounter challenges that will require you to be strong enough to get to the end. Those challenges will need your mental strength and resilience, that is why you have to be prepared and set up a way to overcome this.

It can be frustrating or daunting when you meet a challenge, but it is important to remember not to dwell on that problem and instead find ways to get through that hurdle. It is imperative to divert those thoughts of despair or disappointment to something positive to allow you refocus on to the new routine you have.

If it's because your results are not coming, find a way to change things around to allow you to get back on track. Find a coach if you have to, there are a lot of online coaches or within your locality. Your self-discipline will be required consistently because it is that one secret that will make you unstoppable and achieve your set goals.

Include some personal development in your schedule like listening to something positive in the mornings or at night before you go to bed. Let it be something that will speak to you and inspire you to keep on pressing forward. It maybe a podcast, audio book or just read a book. Make it work for you, either read a chapter or such and such numbers of pages per day. This will be gold for you.

Remember that we become what we focus on every day and the greatest gift you you give yourself is your own personal development which no one can take away. Having a strong personal development gives you mental strength and you become an assert to others too!

What To Do When The Habit Is Not Sticking

Starting a habit isn't always easy. Even if you have the strong desire to create an exercise habit, if you don't approach it with the right mindset, personality, it can be quite difficult.

And let's be completely up front and say that sometimes even if you think you have a handle on creating a strong exercise habit, it might not work out. That's okay. There are some steps you can take to figure it out and move forward.

• Ask yourself WHY? Why aren't you able to follow through and create the habit that you want to create? For example, maybe you thought that training for a marathon was going to be the motivator that finally got you out the door and running every day. You found a marathon training plan and started following the program

• Maybe one day you got too busy to run or you got hurt or sick. One day off turns into two and then suddenly you're a few weeks behind in the plan. What happened? Maybe the marathon training motivator wasn't the right plan. Or maybe nothing happened and you're being too hard on yourself and you can pick back up where you left off and continue moving forward with your exercise habit.

• Assess what does work. Examine habits that you've been able to make work. What do they have in common? Why do they work for you when other types of habits don't? For example, maybe you have an excellent habit of putting things away where they belong right after you use them, but you can't create an exercise habit.

Maybe the reason you can put things away is because that habit is simple. Perhaps your exercise habit is overcomplicated. Look for links in your successes because they can tell you a lot about how to succeed with other desirable habits.

· Try something different. If what you tried isn't working, try something different. Maybe you've always tried to train for events and that never works. Instead, why not give variety a try or do something that's fun.

THE FIRST STEP IS OFTEN the most important but it isn't something to ponder for weeks on end. Make a choice. Decide what you want to do and get started. Create a plan and follow through. Also consider that your approach may be a combination of tactics covered in this book.

For example, maybe you train for an event but you train for it in small steps. Maybe you set a huge goal but you work toward that goal with a group of friends. Creating an exercise habit may not be simple, but it's worth the time and attention. Find what works for you and stick to it.

Remember, as I said earlier, mindset is everything. Everything affects everything and the way you speak to yourself about what is happening also affects your results.

CONCLUSION

Life is a combination of challenges and transformation that we encounter every day in our own ways. One of the most important things we can do in this life is to strive towards improving ourselves. But doing so, we give ourselves the chance to attract and influence others to do the same.

There is nothing more pleasurable than seeing yourself achieving what you set out to do! The fact that you have been through challenges and conquered them to see the results makes it even better. Fall in love with your new routine, make it enjoyable and find ways to have fun while doing it. If by any means you start to feel like you don't want to go out and do something, then look at the routines you have in place, juggle them around and find something different to do BUT for goodness sake don't stop.

The idea is to build and master that routine habit first and once it's establishes and in place, you can start to look for the results and you'll find them. Believe me, once you've started and remained consistent your results will begin to show up and you'll wonder why you didn't start sooner. The feeling is incredible, I know it because I have been on the same journey and it's the best gift you can give yourself!

Never forget that this is your own journey and you don't need permission from anyone to begin. You start because you want o change something in your life and become your best version. Many will not understand you or what you're doing it and it's okay, they don't have to understand. It's your journey anyway so you should keep going and moving forward to give dreams a chance to come true.

Always have a reason and motivation for why you're doing what you started. When you have that, you will get fired up each time because you know your goal. I cannot emphasise this enough, start small and build that habit into your affordable manageable routine. I can guarantee to you that when you have this set up, you'll definitely achieve your goals if you don't give.

The most vital thing is to decide what what you want to do, then take the first step towards it and watch and enjoy your journey. You have started that process now by reading this book and it's a great start!

Like one of the greatest speaker of our time Jim Rohn said, *"For things to change you have to change, and for things to get better you have be better."*

———————

———————

Now, what are the most important things that you should be taking away from this book that will stay with you the rest of your life and actually help you on the road to achieving your goals? Without using the obvious answer of *'everything'* there are a few things that are really important to take note of.

First, you don't have to use everything in this book, and you don't have to use it exactly the way it is arranged. Everyone's style and personality is different I said in the beginning and everything listed here may not work for you exactly the way it might work for me. A good example of this maybe the goal system criteria we used earlier. Some people find it hard to set goals or even make it SMART and they prefer the conventional LONG-TERM/SHORT-TERM style of goal setting and then work how to develop habits from those goals.

It is also important to remember that if you have never tried to develop these kinds of habits before, it is going to be a challenge and there are going to times that you fail. This is perfectly normal. Just remember, a failure only stays a failure if you don't learn something from it.

Finally, always remember that you have the ability to be successful at anything you do if you don't give up. Just believe in yourself and start small where you at. Every single successful person in this world who has done what you want to do, began with the same journey that you are about to take right now; setting their first goals and developing solid habits that they did every day to achieve them. You can do the same. All you need to do to be on your way to completing the journey is **take the first step**.

———————

THANK YOU AGAIN FOR purchasing this book! I hope this book was able to help you to see that anything is possible if you put your mind to it and set a plan for success from the start. Good luck with your journey, believe in yourself and stay focused on the price!

Stephen-Jones

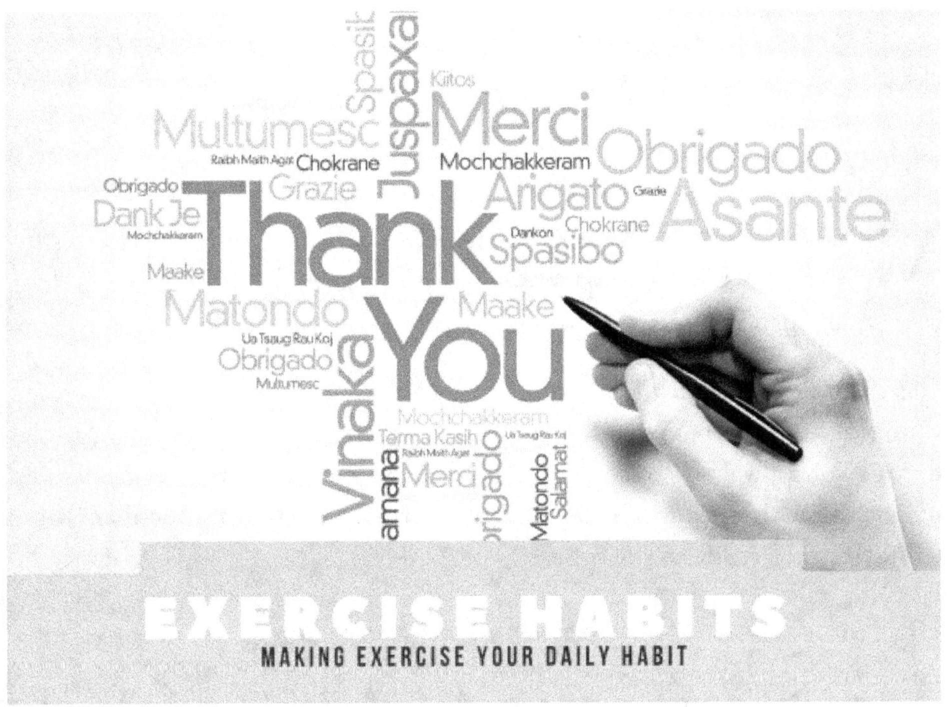

Finally, if you enjoyed this book, then I'd like to ask you for a favour, would you be kind enough to leave an honest review for this book? It'd be greatly appreciated!

Click HERE[1] to leave a review for this book on **Amazon**!

Thank you again and good luck!

If the links do not work, for whatever reason, you can simply search for this title on the Amazon website to find it.

---

1. https://www.amazon.com/How-Make-Exercise-Habit-Happen-ebook/dp/B0874SCL3T

Bonus: Subscribe To The Free Personal Development Resources...

When you subscribe to Your Mastery Life[1] via email, you will get access to free access to exclusive subscriber-only resources. All you have to do is enter your email address to get instant access.

These resources will help you get more out of your life – to be able to reach your goals, have more motivation, be at your best, and live the life you've always dreamed of. I always try to add new resources to the page as often as I can to help individuals which you will be notified of when it happens as a subscriber. **These will help you live life to the fullest!**

Here are some of the resources of what you'll get:

Resilience: Building Your Mental Strength

The Importance of Daily Physical Exercise

How To Practice Gratitude Every Day

Recipes For Healthy Eating

To get instant access to these incredible tools and resources, click the link below:

Click here for Your Mastery Life Resources.[2]

---

1. https://stephenjohnsy.com/home

2. https://stephenjohnsy.com/resources-library

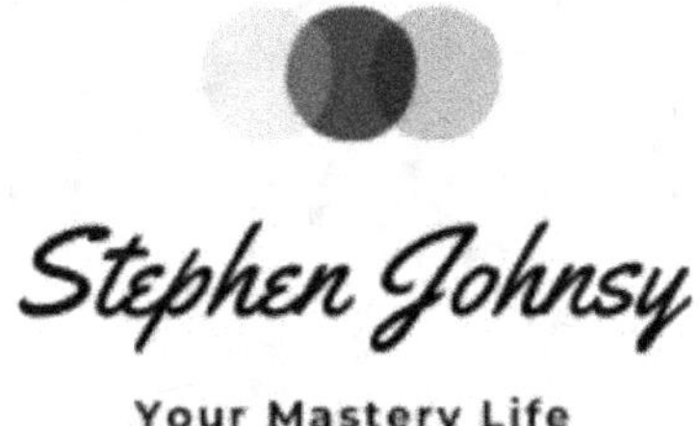
Stephen Johnsy
Your Mastery Life

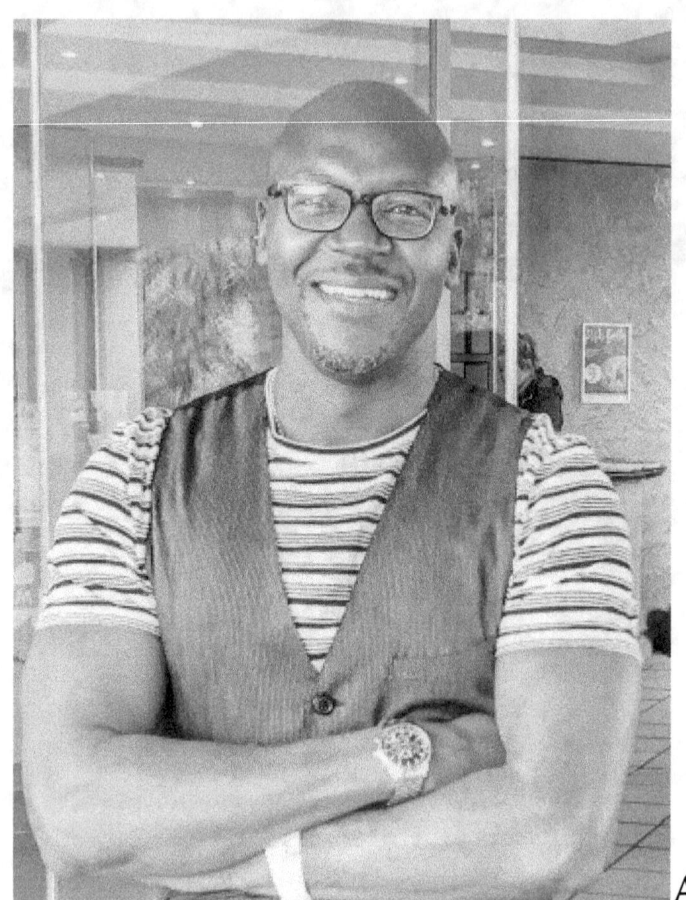

About The Author

Hi, my name is Stephen-Jones Johnson and I'm the founder of <u>YourMasteryLife</u> at https://stephenjohnsy.com[1]. Here is a few words about me.

I am an online entrepreneur, health, wellness, and business coach, a medic and I am passionate about health and fitness including personal development and mindset. I am the founder of YourMasteryLife where I equip, teach, coach, and help inspire men and women around the world on how to live a healthy active lifestyle to reach their full potential with the right mindset and become the best version of themselves.

Through my own personal journey, I have been able to share my own story and in the process find a way to help individuals achieve their own health and fitness results, overcome their challenges to live, and fully enjoy their daily lifestyle.

I am a big believer that personal growth is the key to any progress and success in life and this is what drives me to do what do every single day.

When not writing, blogging, or coaching, I enjoy traveling, listening to classic music, and appreciating nature around me. I believe Life Is A Journey and We Should All Make It Happen For Us by appreciating the little things that come with it!

I encourage you to use my books and linked websites as a resource for you to help set yourself on track to achieve your goals and live the life you and your family deserve and always dreamed of. I have different resources, blog posts, and many more to help you on your journey to better yourself.

---

1. https://stephenjohnsy.com